101 Healthy Living Tips for Business Travelers

101 Healthy Living Tips for Business Travelers

• • •

Robin L. Fleck,

ISBN: 1533499020
ISBN 13: 9781533499028

Disclaimer

• • •

THE FOLLOWING VIEWS IN THIS book are those of Robin Fleck. These are based on her twenty years of experience as a road warrior. The intention of this book is to share her stories and struggles with living a healthy lifestyle and what has worked for her. Her views are based on her experience in everyday life, the corporate world, and education.

Contents

Acknowledgments

• • •

I KNOW I WOULD NOT be where I am today without the inspiration and influence of so many people who made an impact on my life.

First, I would like to thank my parents, Robert and Ellen Korby. Your love and support have helped me become the person I am today and inspire me to keep getting better every day!

Second, I would like to thank my son, Michael Long, who has always required me to be at my highest level of energy to keep up with his every desire in life. His overall success has made it all worth it.

Third, I would like to thank my better half, Craig Becker. Your unconditional love and support drive me every day to live my best life, so we can continue to grow our love and our life together. Your pushing me to complete this book has inspired so much more. I love you!

Introduction

• • •

I've failed over and over again in my life, and that is why I succeed.

—Michael Jordan

As a sales executive for over twenty years and spending my entire career traveling and meeting people, I felt a need to write this book to help other road warriors stay healthy, maintain stamina, and be as productive as possible. I usually spend three to five days a week on the road, and I know from my travels that there are lot of us who live this schedule. This life does not lend itself to living a healthy lifestyle.

I have always been passionate about health and wellness, and I owned two Curves fitness franchises with over fifteen hundred members between the two locations. I ran my organization while still finding time to coach people with diverse needs—from those who were extremely overweight, to those who had recent knee-replacement surgery, to gastric-bypass patients. You name it—I have counseled and worked with individuals on nutrition and exercise programs specific to their unique situations. I am truly driven to help people get healthy.

My passion for health and wellness inspired me to write this book: I realized that the way to reach the most people is not to own another gym or offer more personal training, but to provide easy, healthy solutions for the road warrior.

I want to share my knowledge and experience to help people conquer challenges specific to their health and wellness while regularly traveling for work.

Therefore, this book is the culmination of tips and tricks I have learned over the years while spending 180+ days a year in hotels, airports, and cars. My tips come from both my successes and my failures while on the road.

Over my twenty-year sales career, I have gone from being in the best health of my life to being in the worst health of my life and everything in between. I have bounced up and down twenty to twenty-five pounds many times over the course of my career and my life, so I understand the difficulties of maintaining a healthy lifestyle while dealing with the stresses of travel and work.

I fight my weight every single day. I monitor everything I put in my mouth. That is just the way it is for me, but my health is so important to me that fighting every single day is worth the effort. So even when I fail, I get up the next morning and I start over. If I fail that day, I get up the next day and I start over.

Living healthy is a constant struggle for most of us. We must be aware of our health every day. We must be committed to loving ourselves every day. We must challenge ourselves every day. We must take ownership of our life, every day!

Thank you for purchasing my book. I hope you find it entertaining, informative, helpful, and possibly the first step in living healthy for the rest of your life!

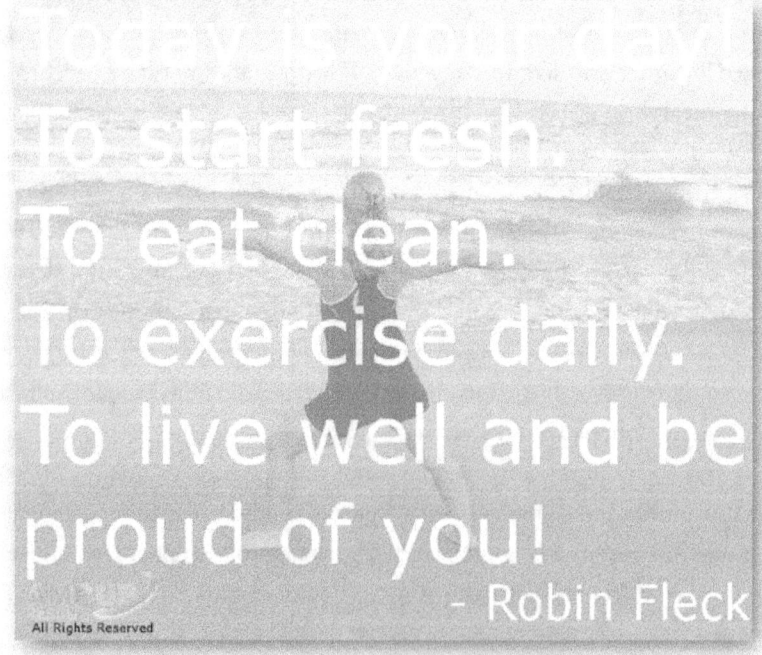

CHAPTER 1

Packing

● ● ●

Why do I always remember the things I forget?

—KEITH BECKER

AS A BUSINESS TRAVELER SPENDING 180+ days a year on the road, I had to learn how to pack professionally, effectively, and healthily for trips.

Packing doesn't appear to fall under health and wellness, but packing can cause a lot of stress and be a daunting experience. What you pack can also determine how healthy you are going to be while away, so here are some tips that keep me going stress free and healthy every week.

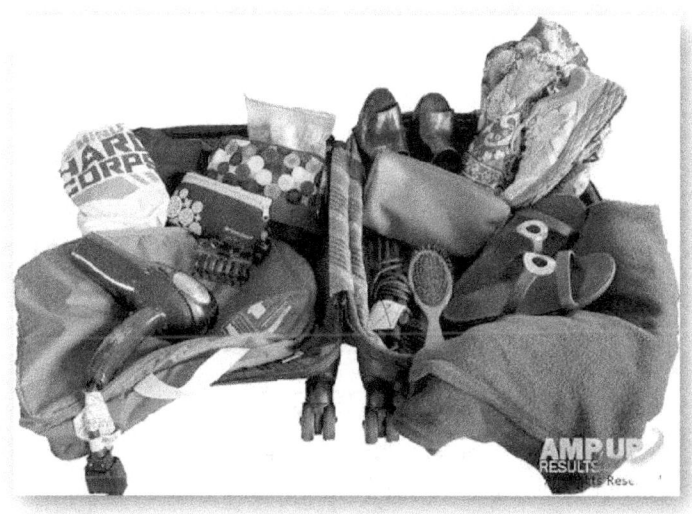

Tip #1: The Ready-to-Go-Bag

In addition to my primary suitcase, I always have a bag of essentials packed and ready to go. This saves me from gathering them up for every trip, and I can concentrate on packing the clothing I'll need for this particular journey.

- Deodorant
- Travel size everything (three-ounce bottles of shampoo, conditioner, toothpaste, hair spray, mousse)
- Hairbrush
- Makeup
- Bar soap
- Travel umbrella
- Neutral-colored scarf
- Airplane blanket
- Cotton swabs
- Cotton balls
- Razor
- Hairclips

Tip #2: Pack a Hair Dryer

Invest in a high-quality travel hairdryer if you have long and/or thick hair that takes a long time to dry. Hotel hairdryers are never dependable.

Tip #3: Packing List

Creating lists removes the guesswork and stress from packing. If you invest 30 minutes creating all your lists, you will save that time and more when you use them later to pack quickly and efficiently.

Tip #4: Use Your Agenda to Pack

Print the agenda for your upcoming travel and adjust your packing accordingly. For example, playing golf with clients will require different gear than attending a black-tie event. We only have to show up once to a black-tie event wearing golf spikes to understand what that does to a dance floor. Lesson learned!

Tip #5: Roll Your Clothes

To save space and reduce wrinkles, neatly fold each item of clothing then roll it into a cylinder before placing it in your suitcase. This practice reduces the amount of air in a suitcase, and air equals wasted space. Using this trick, I can fit a week's worth of clothes into a carry-on and a backpack.

Tip #6: Everything on a Single Hanger

Put your suit, shirt, pants, jacket, belt, ties, etc. on a single hanger. Fold all these items like a shirt and lay on top of everything else in your bag. When you get to the hotel, just remove this from your bag and hang in the closet. Voila!

Tip #7: Spacepak Packing System

The spacepak packing system is a separate set of bags used to organize your clothes to fit efficiently into a carry-on bag or suitcase. The bags come in many sizes and colors.

You can easily get an entire week's worth of clothing into a single bag. It has a side for clean clothes and a side for dirty clothes.

You can view the system at Flight001.com/spacepak.

Tip #8: Flip-Flops

Flip-flops are essential in a hotel room. They take up very little space in your luggage and are a lifesaver for the occasional dirty shower floor or stained carpet. Flip-flops also make that essential coffee run or quick trip to breakfast easier than hassling with shoes.

TIP #9: AIRPLANE BLANKET

I am often upgraded to first class, but this does not happen every time. Therefore, I always pack my own airplane blanket.

Airplane blankets are small yet very warm. They are perfect on the plane and make for a cuddling buddy under the sheets at the hotel.

When the blanket gets worn or dirty, I just swap it out on my next first-class flight.

TIP #10: MOBILE OFFICE

I often have to work from my hotel room in the morning or evening. I want to be comfortable, so I put a lot of thought into what electronics I will need and how to efficiently pack them.

I take my work laptop, a tablet, two phones, and my new watch. I am a technology geek. I move any personal files I might need to the cloud (Dropbox, Google Drive, etc.) before my trip.

Pack a power strip. There are never enough outlets to charge all your devices. Some small-factor power strips are available that allow many devices to be plugged in at the same time.

TIP #11: SNEAKERS

Never forget to pack your favorite pair of sneakers. Your schedule will include a daily workout, but sneakers are also great for wearing before your meeting or walking the long distance to your conference booth. Pack your sneakers in a separate shoe bag for easy swapping with your dress shoes right before you go into your meeting or arrive at your conference booth. This way you avoid ruining your day with sore feet.

In addition, you can attach your shoe bag to the outside of your backpack with a carabiner. This will keep your dress shoes and sneakers in shape and keep your backpack from having a bad odor. Just kidding!

Tip #12: Workout Clothes

Always pack some sort of workout clothes, depending on what you have sched-uled. Here is my list of workout gear:

- Running shorts
- Sports bra
- Tank top
- Sweatshirt/Jacket
- Workout shorts
- Sneakers
- Running belt for room key and phone
- Swimsuit

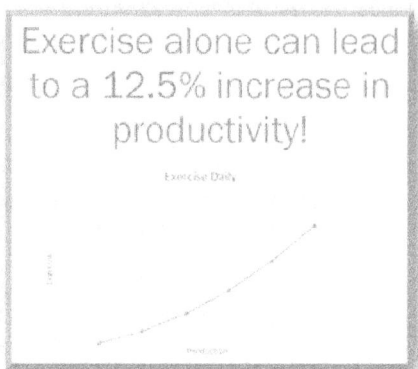

Exercise alone can lead to a 12.5% increase in productivity!

Tip #13: Backpack

I believe top-end designers and chiropractors are in cahoots. Our bodies are not designed to carry bags on a single shoulder, so stop carrying every-thing this way. No one is looking at your stylish bag, but people are prob-ably looking at your abnormally curved spine. Gentlemen you might not go for the top designers but I have seen you with heavy bags, and you need a backpack, too!

Use a backpack and wear it over both shoulders when you have a long walk.

Tip #14: Coordinate Your Layers

When planning your list and agenda, make a conscious effort to wear all the same color. Trying to pack a black, a brown, and a navy suit will overload your suitcase just with shoes. Pack one color of suit, with a single pair of shoes and belt. Pack multiple tops or dress shirts in different colors, and include your preferred accessories.

Tip #15: Photos of Important Documents

Make sure you have a picture of all your important personal documents in your phone and saved to your cloud drive (e.g., Dropbox, Google Drive). This allows you to retrieve important information if misplaced or needed while traveling. I learned this lesson the hard way. I was pulled over in Phoenix for running a red light—"I swear it was yellow"—and in my normal everyday fashion I argued with the police officer. He asked for ID and insurance card, and of course I had my ID, but I never carried my insurance card. It is illegal in most states to drive without your insurance card and they can confiscate your vehicle. Lesson learned. Lucky for me, hubby was available to send me a picture of our card, and now I have everything in my phone in an album.

* Driver's License
* Passport
* Global Entry Card
* Credit Cards
* Car Insurance Card
* Health Insurance Card

Tip #16: Extra Undies

I almost always check my bag with the airline because I usually connect from a small plane in Charlotte, and too many times I have missed my next flight while waiting for my bag. Packing extra undies in your carry-on is vital. If your flight is cancelled, or your luggage is delayed, and you are in a city for an extra night without your luggage, an extra pair will make sure your morning is a little fresher.

Tip #17: Enroll in Global Entry

Your time is money. I have heard so many times, "My employer won't pay for it," and/or "It takes too much time." Both scenarios are just excuses. Initially enrolling in the programs does cost money and time; however, long term it saves you an abundance of both. Recently, TSA has been all over the news for three-hour wait times in security lines in all the major airports. I was at one of those airports—I walked to the pre-check line and was through in less than fifte minutes. When you are on a strict schedule of meeting clients and wanting to get home, it is not worth any amount of money to be delayed over something you can't control. Whatever it takes for me to get home on time is worth the money!

To enroll in Global Entry, visit GOES-app on the web and choose Global Entry from the Trusted Traveler Programs menu.

Tip #18: Always Wear a Scarf

Scarves are perfect for many reasons. They are thin and light, making them easy to pack. They are beautiful, can accessorize any outfit, and give you an overall polished look. You can even roll one up and use it for a pillow on your flight.

Tip #19: Jump Rope

Packing a jump rope is easy. Remember how much fun we had jumping rope as a kid? Doing it as an adult is highly recommended and beneficial because it burns more than 10 calories a minute while strengthening your legs, butt, shoulders, and arms. You can burn more than 200 calories in two ten-minute sessions each day.

When you jump rope, make sure to shorten the rope so the handles reach your armpits while standing on it with both feet and wear properly fitted sneakers.

Tip # 20: Your Phone = Navigation System

This was not a tip I would have thought to add, but on several recent trips I was with other sales executives who all had Garmin or TomTom navigation devices. This surprised me, as I had been using Google Maps on my phone for years— using an actual navigation device just means more to carry and more frustration with connection times and incorrect directions. Most of us already have a phone and Google Maps, so why not use them to get around?

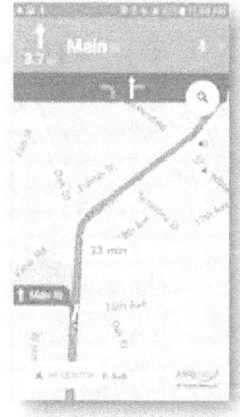

CHAPTER 2

Travel Entertainment

● ● ●

Maybe entertainment is not supposed to be reality.

—Victoria Jackson

Technology has certainly changed our travel entertainment options over the years. We have up-to-the-minute news information on our phones, access to millions of movies and television shows, and apps to relax us, energize us, and even entertain us.

I enjoy using the time on a flight to be entertained. It is the only time I have an excuse not to have my phone on and be connected. I actually relax and enjoy the freedom of flying. My moods and interests are always changing, so I have a wide variety of tips in this section.

Tip #1: Noise-Cancelling Headphones

A flight life-changer. This is a purchase I had put off for years. I thought they looked funny, and I was worried about messing up my hair. How ridiculous! After being frustrated by not being able to hear a movie on a plane with my regular ear buds, I purchased a pair of the Bose Noise-Cancelling headphones. Hello, heaven! I no longer hear outside voices or crying babies when I am trying to read, watch a movie, or sleep. An absolute must-have!

Tip #2: Subscribe to Paper Magazines

Paper-magazine subscriptions are inexpensive and the magazines themselves provide hours of entertainment while traveling. Find some that meet your varying interests, and avoid being bored with just a single topic.

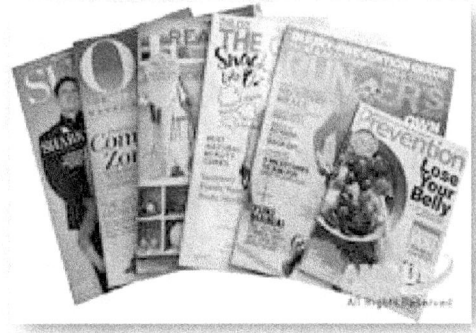

On short flights, long tarmac waits, and layovers, you will be more likely to read a quick article than open a novel. You also do not have to pull out your electronic devices and be logged on.

When I am finished with a magazine, I often leave it in the terminal or in the seatback pocket for someone else to enjoy, but I make sure to tear off the address label—I do not want uninvited guests showing up at my house!

I subscribe to these magazines:

Entrepreneur	*Success*
LiveHappy	*Oprah*
Women's Health	*Dr. Oz*
Fitness	*Runner*
Real Simple	*Self*

Tip #3: Snap Pictures

Create an album on your phone and take pictures of interesting images, articles, and advertisement from the magazines. This helps provide ideas for posting to social media and creates my shopping list for things I want to purchase. Everything is organized in one easy-to-access location. Once I use the information, I delete the picture.

I used to rip the pages out of the magazine, but this just led to large piles of paper on my desk, kitchen counter, and nightstand that I never looked at again.

Tip #4: E-Reader

If you have heard people talk about the Kindle but haven't tried one yet, perhaps it's time to try one. If you have a stack of books you're trying to get through, having them all loaded on your e-reader allows you to change from book to book without carrying the weight.

Amazon's Kindle Unlimited program allows me to have ten book titles available to read at all times. I make sure to have two new books on every trip: one on professional or personal development and another for pure reading enjoyment.

You do not need to have a Kindle Reader to enjoy this Amazon feature. Almost any device can now download the Kindle App that can access your Kindle Unlimited books. If you're like me, you relish catching up on your reading during a long flight. The peace and quiet of a flight without a cell phone is the perfect opportunity to enjoy time to yourself.

Tip #5: Download Audiobooks

If you don't like to read, audiobooks are an alternative—they are a easy way to get through the stack of books you have been wanting to read. I also enjoy listening to them in the car while I am driving to all my locations, when physically reading isn't possible. Try Audible online to find the widest selection of audiobooks.

Tip #6: Download Movies

Not all streaming services are created equal. Netflix does not allow downloading of any movie or television show for later viewing. Amazon Prime Video on the other hand does allow you to download movies and television shows onto a Kindle to watch at your convenience.

I travel with one movie and one television series on my Kindle. This way I can watch a quick episode of *The Newsroom* (an awesome series that should never have been cancelled) for that thirty-minute hop or an entire movie for that Charlotte to Vegas marathon, which I do way too often.

Flight time is my TV time. I do not watch television at home, except for sports. I find watching a TV show or movie can help change my mood and get me ready for my crazy schedule to come.

Tip #7: Bring Your Journal

Flight time is a quiet time to write about the feelings I don't express openly; writing them down and thinking about them helps me feel better and more confident about whatever situation I'm currently handling in my life. I also like going back and reading these entries to get perspective on how things have changed since I wrote them.

I also keep a gratitude journal, something I strongly believe in. I try to write about gratitude or list several things I am grateful for every day.

Tip #8: Coloring Book and Pencils

I haven't started carrying these with me on a plane; however, they are the hottest thing right now for adults seeking relaxation, so don't be afraid to pack them in your carry-on. Coloring allows our minds to wander and reminds us of when we were children.

Tip #9: Download Games

I am not a big game player, but most people around me are heads down into their games, so load a few on your phone or tablet and don't be ashamed to engage in a little fun competition.

Tip #10: Phone as Organizer

Use this time to organize your life in your phone. Create your to-do lists, make photo albums and organize your pictures, create e-mail folders, and file things appropriately.

CHAPTER 3

Snacking

● ● ●

If you get the inside right, the outside will fall into place.

—ECKHART TOLLE

WE HAVE TO BE BETTER at eating what fuels us and in the correct portions. This is especially true when traveling; our bodies are tired, which causes us to crave more sweets and bad carbs, but sweets and bad carbs make us more tired and feel hungry faster. It is a vicious cycle. Bad carbs tend to be sugars, the type of processed or refined food that breaks down easily in the body, which gives you a quick peak or a sudden jolt of energy and then a crash.

I try to live the same way on the road as I do at home. You cannot alter your eating habits or workout schedules just because you are on the road. Health and fitness is a way of life, not a temporary situation.

Make sure to pack your own snacks for the trip. This will allow you to feed your cravings and still make healthy choices.

Eliminating unhealthy carbs from our diet is so important, but especially when traveling. This means SUGAR! Sugar causes our bodies to react in negative ways that reduce our stamina, concentration, and energy.

TIP #1: PREP AND PACK ALL YOUR SNACKS

When I'm home, I prep all my food for the week, and I do the same if I am traveling. I use snack-size bags and cups. Packing everything in portion-controlled containers creates your own single-serve grab-and-go snacks. I use cups for pumpkin seeds because they are perfect for a single portion. I use snack bags to store the single serving of nuts I eat each day (almonds, pistachios, and walnuts).

TIP #2: MEAL-REPLACEMENT BARS

I am not a huge fan of meal-replacement bars; however, I never leave home without them. They can be a savior when there aren't many other options and you are on a tight schedule. Don't fall into the "healthy bar" trap, because there really is no such thing. Look for brands without additives, choose whey over soy, and look for 100% protein concentrate, not isolate.

Atkins bars are my usual choice. They are high in protein and fiber, low in sugar and carbs, and taste good. Atkins provides many options for snacks and/or meal replacements.

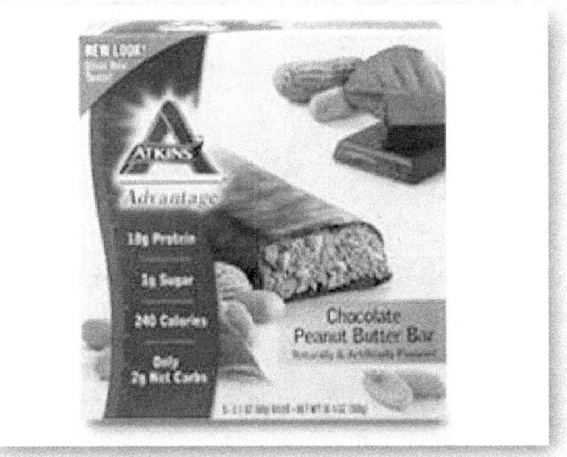

Atkins Chocolate Peanut Butter Bar

TIP #3: PROTEIN SHAKES

There are a lot of protein shakes on the market. I never liked any, or even the concept of them, prior to finding Shakeology. Depending on the flavor, a shake can contain as little as 140 calories and all are packed with the highest quality protein. Shakeology says their shakes are "your daily dose of dense nutrition" because they are packed with so many nutrients. Hundreds of doctors, scientists, and food experts have evaluated the ingredients and have found it to increase your energy and stamina, improve your digestion and regularity, reduce junk food cravings, and assist in weight loss. Shakeology isn't inexpensive, but when I factor in how much I spend on my daily diet, and I usually have this as a meal replacement, it is well worth the cost. I never leave home without packing one per day.

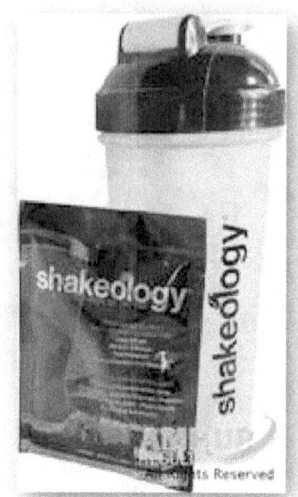

Shakeology helps reduce my junk-food cravings, provides healthy energy, and supports my immune system. It has no artificial flavors, colors, sweeteners, or soy.

And when I am home, I use it to make some very yummy desserts.

Tip #4: Love Hummus

Hummus is my new go-to snack. It's a spread or dip made from chickpeas (garbanzo beans), which are low in fat and carbohydrates, have no cholesterol, and are moderate in protein. Hummus is sold in individual portions that do not require refrigeration. Look for them in the chip aisle of the grocery store.

Make sure you eat the hummus with some raw veggies—avoid pretzels or other high-calorie, high-carb snacks—or you can just eat it with a spoon. Flavored hummus (red pepper, pine nuts, and others) are healthy choices as well. Use hummus in place of mayo or cheese on a sandwich.

Tip #5: Airport Fruit

You can now purchase bananas, apples, and cups of grapes at almost every store in an airport. I prefer to purchase them versus pack them so they do not get damaged in my bag—I do not like bruised bananas.

Tip #6: Bring an Empty Water Bottle

Water is the most important of anything we put in our body. Water can have a positive or negative impact: too little equals dehydration, too much equals bathroom trips, just right equals happy cells and healthy skin.

However, if you ask me this at 5:30 a.m., I will say drink coffee. We will discuss water in detail later in the book, but for now, instead of snacking, try taking a long drink of water to feel full—it may be enough to get you to your next meal without intake of extra calories.

Avoid fruit juices on planes as they include large amounts of sugar and will make you groggy.

Soda, even diet, is never a good alternative. Anything with caffeine can actually dehydrate you more.

Tip #7: Snacks on a Plane

We all love free stuff; however, do not take the snack offered on the plane. If you want to participate and take the snack, put it in your bag immediately and take it home to your kids, but do not eat it! Mindless eating can create unintentional failure. If you are truly hungry, eat the portion-controlled snacks you packed. The snacks on the plane are an extra 150–200 calories of pure sugar and/or bad carbs.

Tip #8: Don't Snack while Driving

Driving can result in mindless eating. Place your snacks in the trunk of the car or all the way in the back of your SUV. Never place them within reach. If they are accessible, you will find and eat them.

Make a rule that you will not eat in your vehicle. If you need a snack or a meal, sit outside or at a restaurant. This will end the mindless road eating that we all find so easy to do.

Tip #9: The Hotel Cookie

310 calories
18g fat
33g carbs
22g sugar
4g protein
Hey, hotels! Where is the fruit?

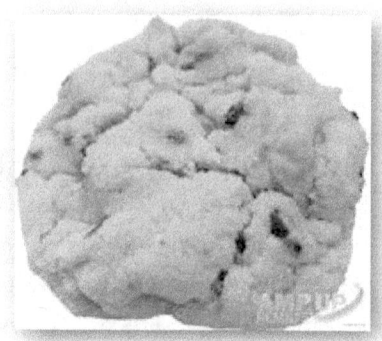

Tip #10: Beware of the Concierge Lounge

I enjoy the convenience of concierge lounges on those nights I don't feel like going out for dinner. Most lounges have healthy alternatives that are the perfect portions. However, enter with a plan because the deep-fried food and the amazing cheese platter can be very tempting.

Tip #11: Mindless Snacking

All of us turn to food at least occasionally to satisfy emotional needs. We eat as a comforting distraction when we are anxious, bored, lonely, angry, or caught up in a wave of confusing feelings. Try to make a conscious effort to think about what you are putting in your mouth before you actually put it in your mouth. The easiest time to eat mindlessly is when we find ourselves traveling alone and we are tired, bored, and exhausted. We must always stay aware!

Workouts

● ● ●

Someone busier than you is working out right now.

—Anonymous

GET UP! GIVE YOURSELF AN advantage and work out! Working out increases your energy and releases endorphins that will make you more productive. Working out on the road can seem impossible at times. Here are a few of my favorite excuses that I have heard (or used):

- I arrived late.
- I do not have my sneakers.
- The gym is probably closed.
- I don't have time.
- I can skip today; I will do butt clenches during the meeting. (I made this one up, but I may try it in the future!)

We must change our attitude about workouts. Your workout should be the same habit or routine as brushing your teeth and you do not go a day without it! As business travelers, we are proficient at organizing our travel and preparing for meetings, so we should take the same care in preparing for our daily workouts.

We all have the same twenty-four hours in a day. You can choose to make your health a priority or not. Make time, not excuses.

Excuses are dream stealers and health killers.

—Brooke Castillo

Tip #1: Schedule your Workouts

Always schedule your workouts into your weekly plan. All my meetings are scheduled and so are my workouts. Also, include any special items you will need for your workout in the notes of your meeting. For example, if a workout requires resistance

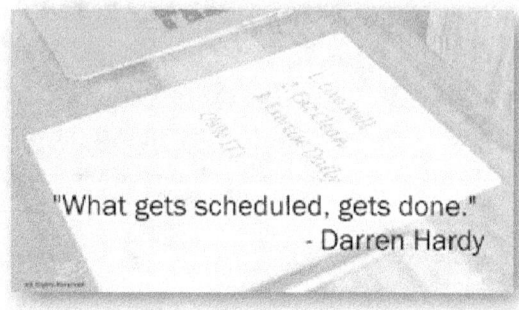

"What gets scheduled, gets done."
- Darren Hardy

bands, include that in your notes. This way, when you pack your bags, you will recognize you need to include your resistance bands.

Tip #2: Check the Gym Hours

I try to stay in a chain hotel that has twenty-four-hour gym access. My days are long and my workouts typically have to be at 5:00 a.m. Whether you are using the hotel gym or a local gym, verify that the hours you scheduled your workout are going to be available when you arrive at your location.

Tip #3: Visit the Gym before You Work Out

Make a quick visit to the hotel gym and test the equipment you are planning to use. There is nothing worse than being prepared to work out and finding out all the treadmills are out of order or they do not have weights as advertised on their website. Yes, this has happened to me more than once. That brings us to our next tip.

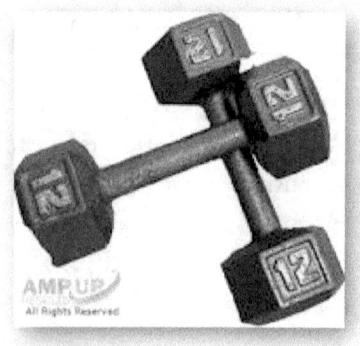

TIP #4: POCKET WORKOUT

Always have a Plan B, or "pocket," workout. Something you can do if the equipment you want to use is out of order or in use. A fun pocket workout is a HIIT (High Intensity Interval Training). With this method, you select four or five exercises that you will do for three or four cycles of one to two minutes each. Make sure to add a warmup and cool down cycle and you are all set! There are thousands of these workouts online—just search for HIIT Workout.

TIP #5: FIND A SAFE PLACE TO RUN

If you prefer running while traveling, determine a safe place to run by doing your homework. Do not take this lightly. Here are a few safety suggestions:

- Ask at the front desk if there is a running area nearby or if the roads around the hotel are safe to run.
- Check online for local running paths before traveling.
- Check online for local running groups and their scheduled runs. Meetup is a great website for finding local groups.
- Schedule runs during daylight.
- Find a mall. Malls tend to be well lit with large parking lots, and they often have twenty-four-hour security.
- Use Google Maps' crime statistics feature to check the areas you plan to run.
- Check the weather before you leave home to make sure you pack the right running gear.

TIP #6: BEACHBODY ON DEMAND

This is my gym membership. You can work out anytime, anywhere with Beachbody on Demand. Stream your workouts to any device wherever you are. There are over four hundred proven workouts to choose from, and you have unlimited access. Visit BeachbodyOnDemand.com for a free thirty-day trial.

If one of the workouts I feel like doing requires equipment, I may use the equipment in the hotel gym or modify the workout to exclude that piece of equipment. Modify doesn't mean skip.

TIP #7: SEARCH ONLINE FOR WORKOUTS

There are at least three dozen workouts online (or maybe more like 3 million). A simple search will give you more results than you could do in a lifetime.

Be specific: if you want to do yoga, make sure to include "yoga" in your search. YouTube is also a convenient source for all types of workouts. Just remember to have a plan. You can spend your thirty minutes searching for a workout and never get to the actual workout. Schedule in advance and know what you are looking for. Once you find a favorite, be sure to save it in your browser for future workouts.

TIP #8: DOWNLOAD A WORKOUT APP

There is definitely an app for that. A workout app can provide any type of exercise you are looking for with step by step instructions and motivation. There are over forty apps for the 7-minute workout alone! The 7-minute workout can be useful when you are limited on time, but it can also be very effective for building muscle and weight loss if you do at least three times through on a regular basis.

There are too many workout apps to list here. Just recognize that if you want to work out, you can find an app to help you.

TIP #9: USE THE HOTEL POOL

This is definitely one place you and I will never meet unless it is poolside, lying in the sun, getting a tan. I have a bit of a public-pool phobia. However, me aside, swimming is a popular exercise, and a bathing suit is one of the easiest and lightest things to pack.

Once again, make sure to check the hotel's pool schedule before adding a swim workout to your schedule. Pool hours are often limited for busy business professionals.

* Sitting in the hot tub kicking your feet with a glass of wine does not count as exercise, but I do not blame you for trying!

TIP #10: LOOK AROUND YOUR ROOM FOR RESISTANCE

If you need weights for a workout, look around your room for objects to help.

- Use a straight-back chair to perform two-arm curls.
- Use your iron filled with water for single-arm curls or presses. Use the two large eight-dollar bottles of water as dumbbells if they are available. Just do not drop them and break them. Make sure to return them to their original location so you don't get charged.
- If you need someone to hold your feet for sit-ups, simply tuck your feet under the couch and crunch away.

TIP #11: 10,000 STEPS EVERY DAY

Getting 10,000 steps every day is important to maintaining a healthy lifestyle. Use a tracking device like a pedometer, Fitbit, or a watch to make sure you are achieving your goals. There are lots of ways to add steps to your daily routine. Use the stairways in hotels versus the elevator. Park your car at the furthest spot in the parking lot. March in place in your room while watching TV.

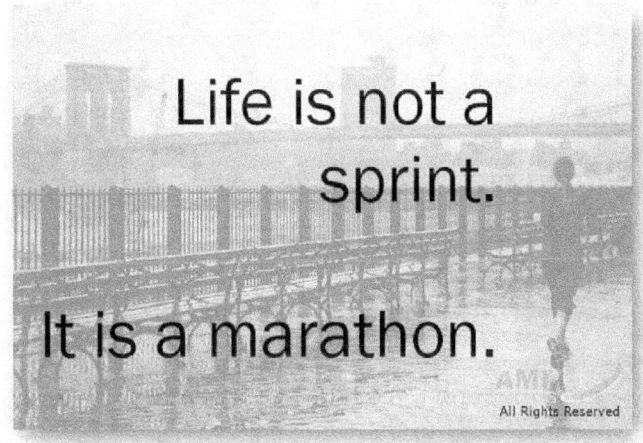

CHAPTER 5

Dining Out

● ● ●

When I eat like crap, I feel like crap.

—Robin Fleck

Maintaining a proper diet while traveling is very difficult. The most difficult part is having to dine out day in, day out. A small per diem, limited options, or being very tired all contribute to making the easy, fast, and unhealthy choice.

Many people want to pocket their per diem. Do not go cheap here. Your health is more important than twenty-five dollars a day. Eating unhealthy at a fast-food restaurant may give you a couple extra dollars in your bank account, but you'll spend them on your copays at the doctor's office. Make healthy decisions.

You must think creatively if your choices are limited. I have included some alternatives in the following tips.

Do not allow being tired to be an excuse for making poor eating decisions. From this day forth, look at being tired as an emotion, not an excuse. We all get tired. We all react differently. Recognize you are tired, but do not allow it to control you.

Tip #1: Choose a Restaurant over Fast Food

Sit-down restaurants can provide healthier food choices than fast-food restaurants. For a few dollars more, you can get a nice salmon or grilled chicken salad or side choices of fresh vegetables that are not lathered in butter or oil.

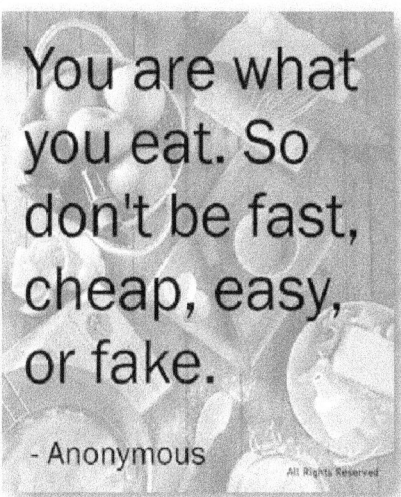

You are what you eat. So don't be fast, cheap, easy, or fake.

- Anonymous

Tip #2: Ask Questions about Food Preparation

Be willing to investigate how specific dishes are prepared. Do not be afraid to ask if they use butter or oil to cook your vegetables. Butter and oil can add a lot of extra calories to your meal without you even knowing. Every restaurant can steam vegetables if asked.

Tip #3: Order Food with Specific Instructions

Now that you know how they are preparing your food, let them know how they can change the food preparation to meet your needs. You wouldn't hesitate to ask at a fast-food restaurant to hold the onion, so don't be afraid to ask at a sit-down restaurant to hold the butter.

Try these suggestions when ordering:

- Ask them to limit the amount of oil used during preparation
- Ask them to not add salt during preparation
- Always ask for condiments like sauces, salad dressing, mayonnaise, and BBQ sauce on the side
- Ask the server for healthy alternatives

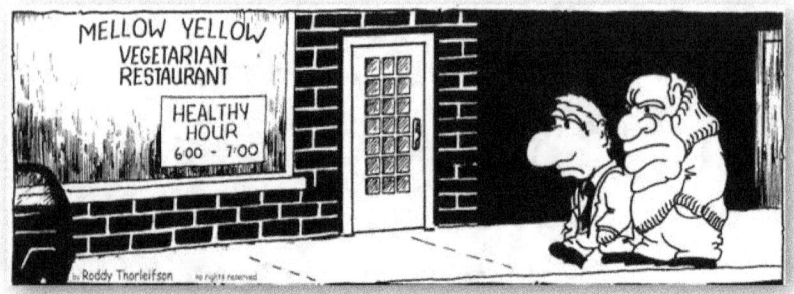

www.mooselakecartoons.com

Tip #4: Order Lean Meats and Fish

Stay with lean meats and fish to reduce fats in your diet. Lean meats include chicken and some types of steaks, like a filet. Rib-eye and strip steaks are delicious but are loaded with fats (probably why they are so tasty!).

These fish are lean:

Bass	Halibut
Bluefish	Mahi-mahi
Catfish	Orange Roughy
Cod	Sea Bass
Flounder	Snapper
Grouper	Tilapia
Haddock	Trout
	Tuna

These fish are fatty:

Carp	Salmon
Chilean Sea Bass	Whitefish
Mackerel	

Even choosing a fatty fish is better than many red meat choices. A salmon salad is one of my favorite meals while on the road.

Also, try to be environmentally conscious when choosing your fish. Ask if the fish is wild caught or farm raised. You always want to eat wild caught fish and preferably from cold waters. Any sit-down restaurant will know where they are purchasing their fish. You can also download the Seafood Watch app to assist with choices.

Tip #5: Don't Eat Bad Carbs

Choose the vegetable side dish over the carb side dishes. Stay away from sides containing potatoes, pasta, cheese, bread, or sugar. Bad carbs enhance jet lag and cause your body to crave more carbs and sugar. Instead, get a second vegetable or a double order of vegetables.

Your server may even know of a special vegetable dish that is not on the menu. Do not be afraid to ask!

Tip #6: Start with Water

Drink water before your meal. This will decrease your appetite, and you can never go wrong with hydrating.

While out with clients, most people will have an alcoholic drink or two. Sipping water while drinking alcohol will decrease the effect of the alcohol, slow down alcohol consumption, and decrease the dehydrating effects of alcohol that are a main factor in hangovers. If you want to feel like you are ordering a cocktail, order a club soda with a splash of cranberry juice—problem solved!

Tip #7: Skip the Bread Basket

Avoiding bread at dinner will help you avoid rolls while sitting at the beach. Enough said!

Tip #8: Always Ask for Dressing on the Side

Be the controller of your own fate. Limit your salad dressing intake by always asking for it on the side. Some salads can have more calories than a full meal when served with the dressing on the salad.

TIP #9: AVOID THE EXTRAS

Sometimes restaurants like to provide you with "extras" beyond your meal. Maybe they will bring out hush puppies or something the cook wants you to try. Try to avoid these. Appreciate the meal you purchased. These are the only calories that you have not accounted for. Free food is not free of calories!

TIP #10: AVOID FAT-FREE AND LITE DRESSINGS

Yup, I said it! Labels can lie. A teaspoon of sugar is fat free. In fact, a fifty-gallon drum of sugar is fat free! Do you see where I am going with this? Many items on the market may be fat free or lite, but are not good for us. Read the label to make educated decisions on what you put in your mouth. Low fat typically means high sugar!

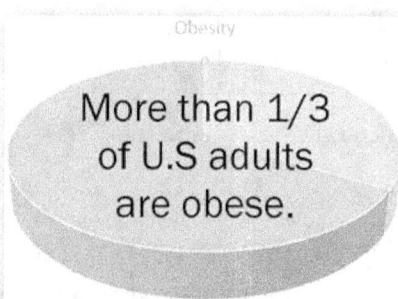

Obesity
More than 1/3 of U.S adults are obese.

TIP #11: LIMIT YOURSELF TO ONE ALCOHOLIC DRINK

You may be surprised to know how many calories are in one beer or a glass of wine. By limiting alcohol to one beer or one glass of wine, we limit our calorie intake and decrease our chances of mindless eating. Further, we decrease our chances of waking up with a hangover.

Waking up with a hangover is a sure way of not working out the next day. Drink in moderation to maintain your health and minimize dehydration.

TIP #12: MAKE HEALTHY CHOICES AT THE HOTEL BREAKFAST BUFFET

Hotels usually offer some healthy breakfast choices. They also offer many poor choices.

Try to choose items that are high in protein and low in carbs like hard-boiled eggs, yogurt, fresh fruit, and oatmeal. When choosing oatmeal, make sure not to add too much brown sugar or dried fruits. Sweeten with Splenda and fresh fruit instead.

Stay away from the carbs. Carbs in the morning will make you fuzzy-brained and make you feel hungry a lot sooner than a high-protein breakfast.

TIP #13: STARBUCKS OATMEAL (WITH A FEW MODIFICATIONS)

I love Starbucks oatmeal with the mixed-nut package and a Splenda. Avoid the dried fruit package, as it is all sugar and very high in calories. Nuts are a healthy, crunchy protein to add, and you might grab a banana and cut it up as well.

TIP #14: SUBWAY

Subway sandwich shops are everywhere and are convenient for a quick, reliable meal. I don't usually choose a sandwich, but I am a big fan of their Chopped Salad. Whether you choose all veggies or add some turkey, it is a healthy lunch, and I find that by adding pickles I don't need any dressing.

TIP #15: AVOID ITALIAN RESTAURANTS

Finding healthy, low-fat options on the menu at an Italian restaurant can be a challenge. If you find yourself in one because the client chose it, ask the server if they serve rice or soba noodles, and always ask for a lower-calorie red sauce instead of a high-calorie white sauce with seafood or chicken. Ask for a double side salad with the dressing on the side.

TIP #16: ASK HOTEL STAFF FOR THE BEST SALAD IN TOWN

I usually ask the check-in staff where I can find the best salad in town. I am not always successful in getting correct information, but it is a conversation starter and they like to converse. You never know what you'll find out about the city your visiting and you might just have the best meal of your life.

Tip #17: Choose Broth-Based Soups

A cup of soup and a salad may sound like the perfect choice, but unless it's a broth-based soup, you're better off without it. Even just a cup of a creamy-milk-based soup is loaded with fat and calories.

Tip #18: Order First

If you are dining out with a group of people, whoever orders first sets the precedent for the rest of the table. If you order a healthier entree, others will follow suit. The opposite is also true. If you order something unhealthy, others will decide one cheat night will not hurt anyone. Be the leader in your group of people wanting to be healthy—make sure you order first!

Tip #19: This is Just another Restaurant

I hear this a lot: "This restaurant is so good and it's a night out, so I should enjoy myself." When you are a road warrior, isn't it always a night out? Doesn't the next town have another highly recommended restaurant? It is important to wine and dine your clients, but let them enjoy their night, you should maintain your healthy lifestyle because there will always be another restaurant in the schedule.

Tip #20: Only Order Dessert for the Client

I discourage the server from even bringing a dessert menu, but some clients really enjoy dessert. If this is the case, pick one for the table and have the server bring many forks. Everyone will be satisfied with a bite, and it is always fun to share.

Tip #21: Order from the Appetizer Menu

When dining alone, most times I will order from the appetizer menu. Ordering from the appetizer menu can get you small portions of some tasty items, and you don't need to worry about extras like sides or bread or salad.

Tip #22: Fast-Food Recommendations

Healthy living entails planning and preparation. If you are going to have to eat at fast-food restaurants, know what you're going to order before you get there. Have one or two go-to items for all fast-food restaurants.

Here are some of my favorites and healthiest options:

Chipotle Vegetarian Burrito Bowl. I typically will order with black beans, a half-order of rice, peppers, mild salsa, lettuce and guacamole. This is packed with protein and fiber and is very filling. You won't miss the tortilla!

Chick-Fil-A Grilled Chicken Cool Wrap. The wrap contains flax and oat-bran flour with 15 grams of dietary fiber. Order without the cheese to eliminate some of the sodium and dairy.

McDonalds Grilled Chicken Sandwich. Only 360 calories and 33 grams of protein, so it is filling. Grab a bottle of water and enjoy.

Panera Bread Mediterranean Quinoa Salad with Almonds. This salad is the perfect amount of calories and protein for lunch and will leave you feeling full and satisfied. Ask for the Greek dressing on the side.

If you like the You-Pick-2 option, the Black Bean Soup and one of the salads is an option, too!

Burger King Garden Grilled Chicken Salad. The trick to eating salad is to make sure you limit your dressing intake. One-third of the package provided is typically the correct amount of calories. Always use regular dressing versus fat free or low fat, which contain extra sugar.

Dunkin Donuts Egg White Flatbread. With 4 grams of fiber and 17 grams of protein it will keep you full. Don't even think about the donuts!

Wendy's Grilled Chicken Sandwich. All fast-food restaurants have a grilled chicken sandwich, so when you aren't sure about anything else, this is a safe order.

Subway Chopped Salad. This has quickly become my favorite go-to when I am traveling. By adding pickles and peppers, there is no need for any oil or dressing. Always add turkey for protein.

If you want a sub, try the six-inch Turkey Sandwich loaded with veggies on Nine Grain Wheat Bread, and hold the cheese and mayo.

Tip #23: Grocery Store

Shop around—food does not have to come from fast food to be fast. Supermarkets often have salad bars, fresh fruit, delis, stir-fry, and sushi.

CHAPTER 6

Hydration

● ● ●

Change your mindset, change your life.

—Anonymous

WATER MAKES UP TWO-THIRDS OF our body. It is involved in every system and every event in our body. Nothing happens without H_2O. For our bodies to function properly, we must maintain hydration. Acknowledging this is the single easiest way to improve our lives. Hydration is that important!

There are all kinds of formulas to determine how much water we should be drinking in a day. A good rule of thumb is one ounce of water for every two pounds of body weight. Another rule of thumb is that after your first bathroom trip of the day, your urine should be clear or pale yellow. If your urine is darker, you probably are not getting enough water.

TIP #1: START EVERY DAY WITH A GLASS OF WATER

Your first action of the day should be to drink an eight-ounce glass of water. I keep a full glass on my nightstand. I do wake up many times through the night and need a sip, but I always drink whatever is left first thing in the morning. Drinking water right away helps you to replace what you lost overnight.

Tip #2: Carry an Empty Water Bottle

There are many sizes and types of easy-to-carry water bottles available. I like to have one that fits in the mesh side pocket of my backpack. Fill it after you pass through security and you'll never be the one stuck on the tarmac for four hours without water. Be prepared!

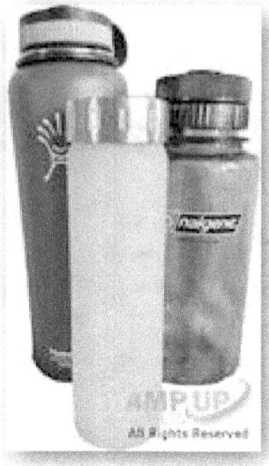

Tip #3: Try Water to Clear your Head

If you are feeling foggy, tired, or emotionally drained, drinking eight ounces of water can truly clear your mind. As you slowly sip the water, your body seems to come back to life. Taking a moment to slow down and drink water has a restorative effect and staves off dehydration.

Tip #4: Increase Water Intake When Your Environment Changes

Working out, traveling, and changing environments can all cause dehydration. The recommended everyday water intake is one ounce for every two pounds of weight, so increase that when you are traveling.

Tip #5: Zero Calorie Benefits of Water

Drinking water naturally suppresses your appetite, helps your body metabolize stored fat, and flushes your system of waste. Drink more water and feel the energy. Enough said!

Tip #6: Stick to the One to One Rule when Drinking Alcohol

Alcohol strips water from the body, so an easy way to prevent dehydration is to alternate between an alcoholic beverage and a glass of water, thus reducing the chance of a hangover.

TIP #7: PREVENT CONSTIPATION

Drinking water assists in digestion and prevents constipation, something we struggle with when traveling.

TIP # 8: ELIMINATE DAYTIME FATIGUE

Drinking adequate water leads to increased energy levels. The most common cause of daytime fatigue is actually mild dehydration.

TIP #9: ALLEVIATE HEADACHES

Water can help prevent and alleviate the headaches we often get from flying or sleeping in a dry environment.

CHAPTER 7

Healthy Choices

● ● ●

The greatest wealth is health.

—VIRGIL

UNDERSTANDING THE NEGATIVE IMPACTS REFINED sugar can have on your mind and body will inspire you to be more careful about the foods you choose.

Understanding the negative impacts bad carbs can have on your mind and body will inspire you to be more careful about the foods you choose.

Understanding how the foods you choose and the activity you do has an effect on your stress levels will inspire you to make better decisions.

Food does not necessarily have to taste sweet to be loaded with sugar. Read labels and beware of convenience and packaged foods. Labels of "low carbs", "low fat" or "diet" should actually be red flags—these labels do not mean free of sugar.

TIP #1: SUGAR PUTS YOUR MOOD ON A ROLLERCOASTER

Unstable blood sugar often leads to mood swings. Sugar causes fatigue, headaches, and cravings for more sugar, all of which contribute to increased stress. Eating a donut at a meeting causes the body to release stress hormones, raises blood sugar, and

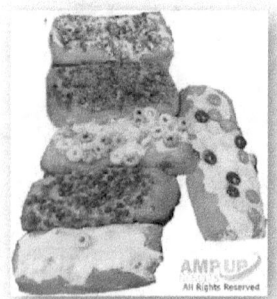

provides the body a quick energy boost. The problem is, the sugar also makes you feel anxious, irritable, and shaky. An hour later you will be hungry and craving more sugar.

Tip #2: Drink Water to Alleviate Cravings

Drinking water and avoiding sugar eliminates cravings and helps you to feel emotionally balanced and energized.

Tip #3: Sugar Contains No Essential Nutrients

People, who eat a lot of sugar fill up on foods high in calories and low in essential nutrients. Eliminating important nutrients from your diet can cause weight gain.

Tip #4: Sugar Suppresses the Immune System

Preventing illness is a high priority in my busy life. I can't afford to be sick while on a trip or get sick and be unable to take a trip. Sugar suppresses the immune response within hours of ingestion, which causes long-term damage to our immune system making you more receptive to the annual flu or cold.

Tip #5: Choose Good Carbs

Carbs provide you the energy and mental awareness it takes to run your life. You will feel confident, alive, energetic, and strong.

You want a well-balanced level of energy that can sustain day in and day out.

Eating good carbs allows your body to process the sugar in a positive way providing you fuel and energy and keeping you feeling full longer.

Good carbs include vegetables, whole fruit, legumes, potatoes and whole grains. These foods are generally healthy.

Tip #6: Don't Choose Bad Carbs

Bad carbs tend to be sugars, the type of processed or refined food that breaks down easily in the body, which gives you a quick peak or a sudden jolt of energy and then a crash.

Eating bad carbs causes inflammation in the body and raises your blood sugar.

Bad carbs include sugar-sweetened beverages, fruit juices, pastries, white bread, white pasta, white rice and other similar processed foods.

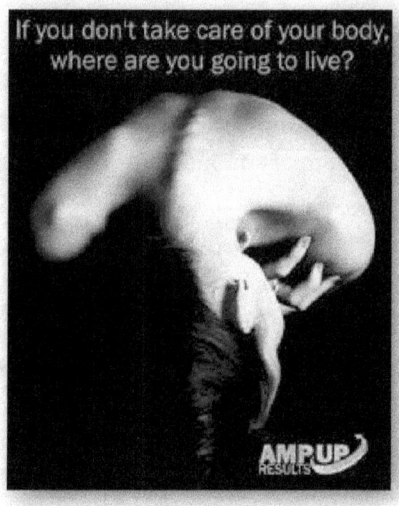

CHAPTER 8

Sleep

● ● ●

Sleep is the golden chain that binds health and our bodies together

—THOMAS DEKKER

PROPER SLEEP IS ESSENTIAL TO maintaining a healthy lifestyle. Research that suggests a major cause of obesity is being chronically sleep-deprived. I have talked to hundreds of colleagues over the years, and most say they cannot sleep well in a hotel room, especially the first night away from home. If you are traveling every week, the first night adds up to a lot of nights, and lack of sleep will do severe damage to your overall health.

Low energy levels from lack of sleep can hold you back. Lack of sleep can cause stress, making you sensitive to small issues and making you become easily discouraged. Lack of sleep causes grumpiness and impatience. This is not a preferred way to have a positive interaction with a client, co-worker, or boss.

The last thing we want to do is exercise when we are tired, but even ten minutes will give you more mental support. It does not matter when you work out; just make sure you get your daily burn. People, who work out regularly sleep better and longer than those who do not.

Sleep is a time of rest and healing that prepares you for the next day's challenges and brings mental focus and consistency.

Proper hours of sleep and quality of sleep will help increase energy levels and cognitive abilities, decrease anxiety and perceived stress, and repair muscles

TIP #1: SLEEP ON YOUR TIME ZONE

Going to sleep and getting up at the same time every day helps set your body's internal clock and optimizes the quality of your sleep. Go to bed at your normal time according to your time zone in order to reduce disruption to your sleep pattern.

TIP #2: USE AN EYE MASK AND EARPLUGS

You never know how loud or how bright a hotel room will be. An eye mask and earplugs can be a savior when you have noisy neighbors.

If you are changing time zones, you may need to rest while the sun is still out and the hotel staff is cleaning or repairing rooms. It is important to get a good night's sleep.

TIP #3: DISCONNECT FROM TECHNOLOGY

Whether at home or on the road, turning off your computer and phone to eliminate their light and sound is essential to how you will sleep. You have to let your body relax and enter a deep sleep in order to get the benefit and restoration. Pinging, dinging, and vibrating phones will never allow you to reach deep sleep.

I know this is hard because we worry about an emergency. I have my phone set up to ring if one of my favorites calls. My favorites are only my husband, mother, father, and son. These are the only people that should be calling me in the middle of the night.

TIP #4: LISTEN TO RELAXING MUSIC

Find some relaxing music that you enjoy, and listen to it before you go to sleep. Comforting music will slow your heart rate and improve your sleep.

Tip #5: Lower the Temperature in the Room

Scientists have proven that lower temperatures are better for sleep. I also like to snuggle up under my covers. This makes me feel more secure and aids in falling to sleep faster.

Tip #6: Sleep with Your Feet outside the Blankets

I am not making this up. Scientists have also proven that cooler feet aid in better sleep! My husband always sleeps with one foot outside the covers. He has always done this, and he never knew why. Recently I read an article that stated sleeping with your feet outside the covers decreases your heart rate and aids in sleeping. I just thought he was weird!

Tip #7: Use a Meditation App

Meditation is a practice of relaxing and restoring the mind. There are many free meditation apps available online. Find one to your liking. Even five to ten minutes of meditation can relax your mind and body. This will put you in the right frame of mind for a good night's sleep. My favorite App is Calm because it has many different sound options and you can choose a guided or quiet meditation.

Tip #8: Tune in to Your Body to Fall Asleep

I am the type of person who falls asleep almost immediately upon hitting the pillow (lucky me); however, I then have a tendency to be wide awake again at 2:00 a.m. Someone told me to stop counting sheep and tune in to my body. Start with your feet and visualize your toes—all ten of them—then move to your ankles, calves, knees, and so on, and by the time you get to your head you will be asleep. I don't know why, but it totally works.

Tip #9: Can't Sleep? Try One Hour of Work or Reading

If you absolutely can't get back to sleep, don't just lie there. Get up and work or read for an hour. The key is to get up, don't just turn on the TV. Getting up and moving around or working will stimulate your body and mind and make your body realize it is still tired so you will be able to lie down and fall back asleep.

Tip #10: Start Walking

A thirty-minute walk in the morning is one of the best ways to get a good night's sleep. Sunlight helps regulate the body's clock and releases mood-boosting serotonin, making you happier through the day and able to rest soundly at night.

Tip #11: Minute Suites

A new concept only available at three major airports enabling you to rent a small, private room with a couch, desk, smart TV and Wi-Fi. This is a great concept when you miss your connecting flight and you don't want to leave the airport to find a hotel. This is the newest **"wellness-based solution to the stress and fatigue caused by air travel"** according to their website. MinuteSuites.com

Bonus Chapter

• • •

THERE IS AN APP FOR THAT!

BELOW ARE SOME OF THE apps I use to make my travel and overall life more organized. I am an Android phone user with an iPad, so these apps tend to play nice across both platforms.

TRAVEL

Tripit. This is worth spending the money to upgrade to the Pro version. It integrates with Concur (if your company is a user), but is much simpler to use, and I have everything I need at my fingertips.

Concur. This is a Travel and Expense application that allows you to take pictures of receipts and track all your expenses. This makes submission of your expense report simple.

Google Maps. I stopped carrying a GPS device a long time ago. Google Maps is the most accurate navigation app I have found, and it has never left me driving into the ocean.

RESTAURANTS

OpenTable. I can always find a restaurant for myself or a group, and making reservations has never been easier.

HappyCow. This app is awesome for locating vegan-food locations. I am not vegan, but I know the food will be healthy. If you are ever in Myrtle Beach, South Carolina, make sure you visit Be Well Meals and Juice Bar.

Starbucks and *Panera*. I use this app to locate the nearest store.

NOTES AND ORGANIZATION

Wunderlist or *Evernote*. I prefer Wunderlist, a simple to-do list with expanded features. Perfect for creating your packing list.

Keep. I like this app to keep my passwords and personal notes, and I do a lot of journaling within Keep.

Trello. Organization for the whole family. Trello is an easy, free, flexible, and visual way to manage your projects and organize anything.

Google Calendar. Having everyone in the family with a Gmail account and a shared calendar can make home life much easier.

FITNESS AND TRACKERS

Beachbody On Demand

  7 Minute Full Workout

  MyFitnessPal, LoseIt, 21 Day Fix Tracker: Food/calorie-tracking apps.

Conclusion

● ● ●

You can have results or excuses—not both.

—Anonymous

As a business traveler spending 180+ days a year on the road and struggling to live an overall healthy lifestyle, it was important for me to share my knowledge and experiences on how I made the decision to take ownership of my life.

The constant weight fluctuation, jet lag, and lack of sleep always made me exhausted on the road and at home. I struggled to find a balance and live my best life while being as productive as possible.

Implementing small changes to my everyday life drastically changed my overall energy, which then changed everything else. I started by focusing on drinking more water and then gradually added all the other tips, like eating at better restaurants, making smarter food choices, committing to my workout, and learning to sleep. The more I changed, the better I felt. I could now fully engage with my clients and build real relationships, giving me a competitive advantage at work and allowing me to spend more meaningful time at home with my family. My overall temperament is better and allows me to focus on the long-term objectives rather than the short-term challenges.

The tips I provided are things I have learned or experienced over my twenty-plus years as a traveler, and my hope is that at least one of them inspires you to implement small changes. If you live a healthier tomorrow than today, and learn to "own it," writing this book was worth it.

If you are interested in more health tips, please sign-up on my website at AmpUpResults.com to enroll in our weekly tips, monthly newsletter or to read my blogs. You can also follow me on Twitter @ampupresults.

About the Author

• • •

ROBIN FLECK IS A MYRTLE Beach–based sales executive, entrepreneur, professional speaker, trainer, one-to-one wellness coach, and road warrior with more than twenty-five years' experience in the financial services industry. She has owned multiple businesses, including two Curves fitness franchises with more than fifteen hundred members between the two locations. Something of a fitness guru, she has also worked as a Zumba instructor, CIZE instructor, and personal trainer. She studied nutrition with the Cleveland Clinic and continues to educate herself through certifications, classes, and self-study. In addition, while she was collaborating with Curves, she mentored women dealing with knee replacements, gastric bypass, obesity, and more. This drove her to become a Certified Wellness Coach and Certified Corporate Wellness Coach.

Robin understands the importance of working with organizations to create a wellness culture that encourages employees to live their best lives. Her company AmpUpResults.com specializes in providing corporations the opportunity to make their employees healthier, increase productivity, reduce turnover, and lower healthcare costs with her highly effective corporate wellness programs. She also provides one-on-one coaching sessions with business professionals and road warriors.

As a professional speaker, Robin is entertaining and engaging in her approach to living healthy. Her passion for sharing experiences and teaching her methodology in a simple and fun way provides audiences everyday tools to living their best lives.

Before she moved to Myrtle Beach, Robin lived in State College, Pennsylvania, and she grew up in Chambersburg, Pennsylvania. She is an avid runner, having completed one marathon and many half-marathons; an active member of the Carolina Boxer Rescue, raising two beautiful boxers of her own; a member of Toastmasters International; and a member of the National Speakers Association. She also trained with Carolina Improv to improve her spontaneity. A mother and a wife, Robin is a family woman with a strong sense of balance in health, fitness, family, and life.

www.ingramcontent.com/pod-product-compliance
Lightning Source LLC
Chambersburg PA
CBHW071124280526
45787CB00003B/1158